FROM ILLNESS TO WELLNESS

I0505626

How I overcame Hypermobility Syndrome – a Chronic Pain Condition and more

Some of the proceeds of this book will be donated to the following organizations: HMSA, GOSH, Arnica and the McIntyre Centre (which provides horse riding to disabled children and young people). All these organisations better peoples' lives.

Note on the front cover drawing: I drew this picture at a very difficult stage in my journey when my homeopath asked me to imagine what life would be like when we were healthy and well again. I looked at it every day to help motivate me. It symbolises strength, wellness, joy and the positive goal of where I wanted to end up. And now I'm here!

I placed drawings by my daughter at different points in the text to open up spaces for your own reflections.

ACKNOWLEDGEMENTS

I would like to thank my daughter, son and husband for helping me and each other out when life was hard because of HMS and forever. My parents for in their own way making it possible for me to get the help I got. 'Old Storm' for looking after me from above; Sigrid too who showed me a better way; Eva and Olivia for your emotional help, care and support; Hypermobility Syndrome Association (HMSA) for teaching me more about HMS and showing me where to begin to seek and get help with referrals and managing Hypermobility Syndrome (HMS); and Great Ormond street Hospital (GOSH) for rehabilitating the kids. Arnica Network, Dawn Waterhouse and Access Consciousness for helping me on the alternative path to health. Debby, Tina and other friends for their support and taking the time to help proof read this book. Andras for helping me publish this eBook. Kurt and all our friends for your friendship and support in the past and present. Young Carers and PALS for being a friend to the kids and all the people and therapists/practitioners who helped my family on our paths to health. At last but not least I want to thank you readers for supporting my journey by reading this book as I hope it'll support and help you on your journey!

CONTENTS

FOREWORD

I am Storm's husband and we have been partners since about 1999. We met in Ireland and I became aware of Storm's Hypermobility Syndrome (to be referred to as HMS from now on) condition pretty soon after we met. To be honest I didn't really understand the full impact of her condition for a while, as at the time she would push herself beyond the pain barriers to try and continue a "normal" life. However, as time passed I began to realise how difficult it was for her to live with HMS. She had already tried various things to lessen or manage her HMS, but little did we know how far she would have to go to lessen and mostly cure her condition. Since we met, we have given birth to two children, got married and in between all that she has tried countless techniques, therapies etc. to lessen the effect of this condition.

You will find this book an interesting and informative read if you want to know what life can be like living with this condition as the sufferer and those that live with a sufferer of HMS. The book also gives some ideas and pointers about what you can do, where you can look and the organizations to consult to work with your own chronic pain condition, whether it's HMS or a similar condition. You will read about the pain, sufferings, heartache and also the successes and hope that can come if you just keep on persisting to find the right answer, whatever that is for you.

If you only learn one thing from this book, then that should be don't EVER give up, no matter what ANYONE says, whether it's family, friends, doctors or professionals. Your solution may not be the same as Storm's, but I believe you will find this a useful resource to begin or continue your road to at least lessening the suffering of whatever chronic pain condition you or your loved ones have.

Good luck and I hope you find the book useful!

Andras Furness

WHAT IS HMS?

Hyper ('too much') mobility ('movement') Syndrome (also called Benign Joint Hypermobility Syndrome or Ehlers-Danlos hypermobility type) is a genetic connective tissue disorder that can affect most if not all of the body as we have connective tissue everywhere. The collagen is faulty i.e. more stretchy than usual, which means the body or the affected parts of the body stretch/give way/move too far so it can cause pains and fatigue as you use your body incorrectly. HMS can cause sprains and breakages easier as the joints and muscles become weak. It is called hypermobility or being hypermobile when you're just extra bendy with no symptoms. When you're extra bendy with symptoms it's called Hypermobility Syndrome. If you'd like to know more about the specifics of HMS you can find it in the books and websites listed in the **Extra Information** at the back of this eBook. As there's a wealth of information on this syndrome and because I found another path to get well, I don't want to get caught up in the scientific explanation too much. I realized recently that it's not as important in the big scheme of things as I once thought it was. HMS is under the banner of Chronic Pain conditions along with Chronic Fatigue Syndrome and Fibromyalgia. They have a lot in common and the treatment at UCL (University College London) Hospitals is very similar if not the same.

These are some of the most common symptoms of HMS:

- Joint pain- chronic/sporadic in one, several or all joints.
- Other pains in soft tissues.
- Headache.
- Fatigue/tiredness.
- Irritable Bowel Syndrome (IBS).
- Anxiety
- Depression
- Heart palpitations
- Easy bruising and more.

I believe everyone has a pre-disposition for some illnesses/conditions in life and I believe various negative influences can trigger them i.e. injury, trauma (mental/physical), too much stress and possibly exposure to chemicals. In our case our pre-disposition was symptoms that showed themselves as HMS.

MY CHILDHOOD AND GROWING UP

When I was a child and very overwhelmed by my symptoms of HMS I very much wanted to write a book about this struggle to let others in the same situation know that there were others out there suffering with the same condition/symptoms. I did start writing it but I then only knew the beginning......now I can finish it as I also know the end......

I grew up in Denmark and as far back in school I can remember I suffered with headaches and lower back pain most days and occasional sprained fingers and ankles. I didn't know at the time it was HMS. The doctor just said it was growing pains........As a 13 year old I went to a boarding school focused on sports and music as I love music and sports and I did every type of sport imaginable. At first I loved it, but as a teenager I was very vulnerable to symptoms of HMS and as I did so much sport my health went downhill quickly after a few months. I was training for a half marathon with the intentions of going on to run a full marathon later but my knees buckled and became so painful that I had to give it up! I was then 14. I gradually was forced to stop doing most sports as the pains everywhere in my body got worse and worse - at times I had to use crutches - and lots of support bandages most of the time. I got bullied by peers and teachers alike as they didn't understand, or believe me, as they saw me walking one minute and limping the next as the pains were intermittent. At the age of 15, I had to stop going to school altogether as I could no longer walk up the stairs to class. It was a very low point in my life and I couldn't see it getting better. By now my doctor had heard of HMS and told me I had it, and there was nothing that could be done about it, no help/cure available and I could never do sport again!

I remember being taken to a rheumatologist who examined me and concluded: "You're fine! There's absolutely nothing wrong with you!" I walked out of there thinking "yay that's great, but why do I still have all these pains and symptoms then?!" I kind of felt like a fraud as the rheumatologist said I was fine, but I said I wasn't (and I wasn't!), but the experts ought to know what they are talking about right?! And they are also the ones most people listen to!

I then went back home to live on the farm in the middle of nowhere with my parents and did not know where to go from there. I was deteriorating and addicted to painkillers by then. The doctor said "you shouldn't be ingesting so many painkillers at your age!" but what could I do?? When you're in severe pain you want it to go away and that was the only way I knew how! By then I also had serious issues with Irritable Bowel Syndrome symptoms such as constipation, haemorrhoids, dizziness, nausea, fatigue and weakness. I felt like I could faint and my knees could buckle at any time. Once on a trip to Sweden I was hospitalized as I felt so bad but as usual they found nothing wrong. HMS was even less known then than it is now. As well they thought something might be wrong with my heart, so they kept me in for observation and did another test in the morning and it turned out to be a faulty machine! One good thing I got out of that trip was a pair of crutches that I used often. But even that was hard as it hurt my hands, elbows and shoulders a lot! Another example of my pains and dilemmas was that I could hardly tie my shoe laces because of pain in fingers and hands. However, I needed to wear that supportive type of shoes as if I chose not to, my ankles, knees and hips would become even more painful!

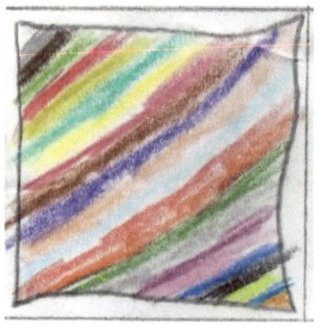

I remember walking and sitting in the countryside thinking and writing on the road 'WHY?', as it was so hard and I really didn't understand why it should be so hard for me?! I was just a teenager who so wanted to have fun and be happy and healthy.

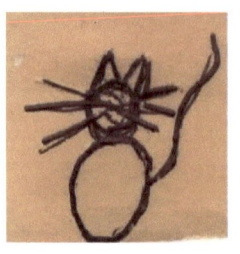

A few months after I came home to live I took an overdose of painkillers one night when my parents went to a party as I'd just had enough! I couldn't do it any more - couldn't live like that any more. I felt like I was hurting my family - bringing them down by being so ill. I felt sick of living as I only got worse and no-one seemed to be able to help. I was desperately lonely as no-one else seemed to know about HMS or have it and most of my friends had disappeared and I thought they probably couldn't stand being around me as I complained of pains and held them back. To be honest I didn't really care if I succeeded in taking my own life or not. On one hand I wanted to die as then all the emotional and physical pain would end, on the other hand if I survived I wanted help!! But I doubted I'd get it as it hadn't happened thus far. I'd even written a suicide letter for my parents to find in the morning! I did wake up again very early after a horrible night of being scared, hardly sleeping, frozen to the spot as I was so scared and hallucinating and imagining the most gruesome things in my head because of the drugs. When I told my parents my mum did call the doctor for help but nothing changed. Then I sort of decided I had to change...and live as if I wasn't in pain as that's what everyone wanted and I couldn't stand living like that any more! So mentally I sort of split myself in two and ignored my pains as much as I could and pretended I didn't have them - even though it felt completely wrong. I dissociated from the pain and decided never to tell my parents if I was in pain again. I couldn't bear the responsibility and guilt I felt from feeling I affected their lives negatively, so when they after school would ask me about my day, I'd say it was all fine!

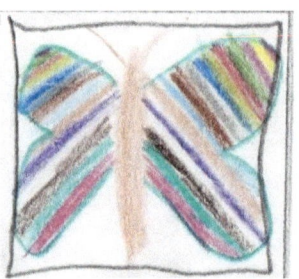

From then on I went back to school even though I'd missed most of a year and I also started singing in a band. After that year I moved away from home at the age of 16 and did two more years of schooling. I was somewhat better as in the months following my suicide attempt my parents took me to an alternative practitioner who helped me via reflexology, healing, talking, homeopathy, herbal remedies and supplements. She was really lovely and very helpful to me. That opened my eyes to the alternative world of healing and medicine.

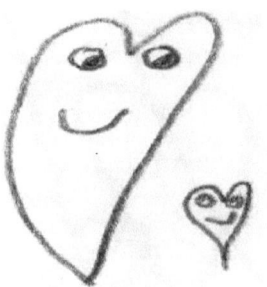

Within those two years I started seeing a psychiatrist as I'd get bouts of depression and since then I've had more than 100 counselling sessions with various counsellors and psychologists - have even studied Level 1 in counselling myself now as I've always known I want to help people some day when I'm well enough!

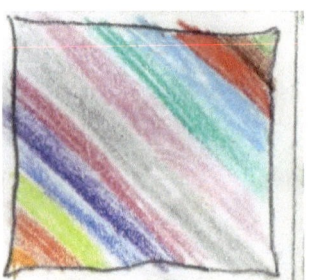

After finishing school I managed to travel and work full-/ and part time, even though at times in a lot of pain. I kept wondering on and off what was going to happen to me eventually...would I one day just break?, fall apart?, never to be able to walk again?...but I kept going regardless as there were nothing else to do. I remember a co-worker telling me that our boss had asked her why I walked so slowly - like an old lady. She'd told him of my condition and he said: "why did she never tell me?", he probably felt deceived, but in those days I felt I couldn't tell employers as then I wouldn't get a job!! Tough situation to be in! I also remember when I travelled with my backpack in London, when I put it on my back and started walking with all that heavy weight my joints and hips would loudly go 'clonk clonk' and I'd walk on in much pain and I'd wonder how it was all going to end?...the only positive side of the way I dealt with it at that time was that I probably kept myself and my muscles strong to compensate for my weak joints which helped me move on (literally and figuratively) by keeping active. Also my attitude of just ignoring the pain and go on regardless didn't feed into a negative thought/emotional cycle (that happened later in my life). It made me better able to go on. Even though none of those strategies were healthy/optimal on their own!

I MET MY HUSBAND AND HAD OUR SON

In 1999 I met my Australian husband in Ireland.
We didn't know that he also had HMS at the time - and
in June 2000 we had our son whilst living in Denmark. I had
many pains during my pregnancy. And even though it was
wonderful to have a baby it was very hard physically as I
struggled carrying and holding him whilst breastfeeding and
carrying auto seats etc. My depression got steadily worse! In
2002 we had a baby girl. We were expecting her to walk etc.
sooner than my son did, as girls often do so sooner than boys
but she was slower...that was my first sign that she might be
affected by HMS. As I knew somewhat more of HMS by
then, I kept an eye out for the signs whilst hoping my
children wouldn't inherit it as my husband was fit and strong
with healthy genes! Or so I thought!! Also when we lifted her
by holding her rib cage below her arms, she'd just slip
through our hands - also a sure tell-tale sign of being
hypermobile to a great extent. All babies are
born hypermobile and that's normal and most become less
and less hypermobile as they grow older BUT some stay
hypermobile and if they get symptoms with it, it becomes
HMS (Hypermobility Syndrome). When my son was walking
as a toddler we noticed he was complaining of pains and
tiredness in his legs, so we took him to a podiatrist and had
special insoles made for both his and my feet when
they measured our feet in various ways. They were really
helpful to wear and he didn't have any symptoms of HMS
again for many years!

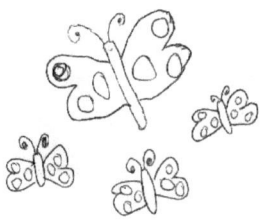

By then I'd decided never to go through the doctors/'system' etc. again as they were never able to help me and it was so hurtful going to see medical specialists who made me feel like I
made it all up as they didn't know what it was nor what to do about it!

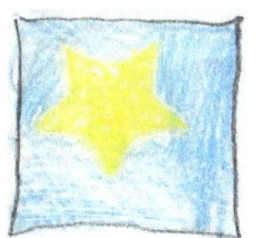

By now I realized I had severe depression. I was prescribed a strong dose of anti-depressants and it did ease my depression - thank goodness! I also started having lots of counselling in a group and one-on-one which was very helpful.

OUR DAUGHTER

I'd had a bad experience giving birth to our son in hospital, so I decided to give birth to our daughter at home in a birthing pool. Even though I experienced much pain giving birth, at least it was in water and at home which was more soothing and the whole experience was much better than in hospital.

We decided to stop having more children partly as I worried that giving birth again would make my HMS worse, as it can do to some people with HMS as the pelvis becomes loose and causes further pain and discomfort.

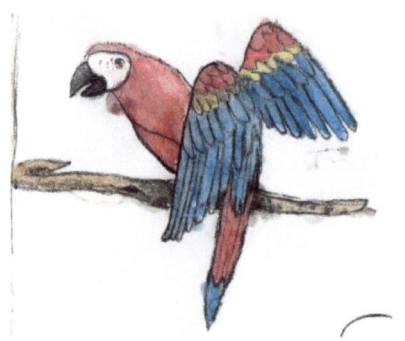

In 2004 we moved to Wales and my daughter would start to display the typical characteristics of a child with HMS: leg pains, fatigue, couldn't walk far, had to take breaks, and didn't want to dance when I took her to toddler music play groups. I tried to get her to see medical specialists twice but because of the paperwork apparently going missing, waiting lists etc. it never happened at that time. In 2008 we moved to Hampshire, England where we experienced a traumatic event as we were harassed severely by our next-door neighbour to the extent we had to flee for our lives. My daughter could hardly walk, so we consulted a podiatrist for insoles, as she was pronating a lot. A rheumatologist referred her for physiotherapy, which also helped. She was in a wheelchair when she started school in England. However with physio exercises and reiki she managed to get out of the wheelchair after some winter months even though I'd been told once you get into a wheelchair with HMS you don't get out again! She received counselling for the traumatic event which I believe caused some of her physical symptoms due to fear she was experiencing. At this time I was in so much pain that I really needed to be in a wheelchair, but it was physically impossible in our house. I also had to wheel my daughter around and open and collapse her wheelchair daily, so I just had to bite the bullet and go on in severe pain! Summers were always best as the pains lessened during the warmer months. My daughter was 7 years of age when another winter came and the pains were very bad. She started crawling again and using walking aids. We had occupational therapists from the council come out to modify the house to assist her in going about her daily routine i.e. a bath pole, better banisters, a bed horse and wall handles for bath and toilet, as sometimes I had to carry her upstairs to use the bathroom as she couldn't get up the stairs!

All the time I kept searching for help as I was desperate and believed help was out there and I didn't want my children to go through what I had gone through as a child. I couldn't imagine them having such a terrible time growing up with pains, other physical symptoms and emotional difficulties as I'd had. I didn't want to accept them having to go through the same pain emotionally and physically. Something had to give, as we as parents were very stressed, in pain and depressed because of the whole situation and seeing our children and each other in more or less constant pain. Our son who was then 9 was now developing serious pains in ankles, knees, shoulders and neck to the extent where he at times used crutches! He also suffered daily from severe dizziness and he couldn't keep up with his homework as he had to help so much with our daughter and do household chores because I couldn't do it all! It was horrible. And my husband spent all his holidays off work on hospital appointments, medical consultations and school excursions, so he also deteriorated physically and mentally!

Through the HMSA I'd heard of some children being referred to Great Ormond St Hospital (GOSH) for treatment for HMS so eventually I got them referred. We all spent 2 weeks there as out-patients where they received treatment such as physio with weights to strengthen their muscles to compensate for their over bendy joints, and also pain management and podiatry. It was hard seeing the kids in even more pain before it got better....but they made it and I've only just recently let them choose themselves when and if they continue to do the exercises or not as they are now so well and rarely experience pains. They are now among the 5% strongest kids in their age group because of the exercises. They are amazingly strong!! That rehabilitation worked well. Their pains lessened and they were able to function without walking aids which was huge for us! It was also good for the kids to see other kids with the same condition and feel 'normal' and accepted and believed at GOSH.

It was a very hard process to go through and they especially my daughter still struggled with pains after the rehab, but they were approximately 70% better than before GOSH! This was a huge improvement for us at the time.

FURTHER HELP/ASSISTANCE WE GOT

During the years 2005 to 2011, I decided to study reflexology as this had helped me previously - also to hopefully help my family's condition, so I became a qualified reflexologist. I also studied aroma therapy, reiki, counselling, holistic therapies and 'first aid homeopathy' as all the above had helped our family improve health wise along the way.
We also had a social worker/family counsellor from the council come out to help us and the kids over several visits and months. I felt my sons dizziness could be to do with stress and anxiety relating to his past experiences and the trauma of having to help too much at home and seeing his family in pain whilst he himself was unwell. And that worked really well. She helped him learn how to cope better, as it was hugely connected and now he's rarely dizzy. She also helped my daughter and me to deal with the pains and gave us tools for going through hard times as we often did on our own, as we didn't really have a network as our families lived abroad and we never really felt accepted in that community, partly as we couldn't really get out of the house much to participate in the community...

After the kids got help I sought help too by daring to go through 'the medical health care system' again, as I'd been so afraid to for years as I had been judged as a hypochondriac when I was younger. Yet I had seen the kids get taken seriously when we went to the right places so I tried also. I got a referral to UCL in London and was re-diagnosed with HMS/chronic pain condition and placed on a course of eight separate sessions in London. The appointments were very hard to get to as I had to travel from South Hampshire on public transport in my bad condition, but I did it as my drive to become well and heal my family always has meant everything to me. The sessions were very helpful and consisted of a mixture of pain management, relaxation, cognitive therapy, 'pacing' and some private psychology sessions. I also went there a couple of times for extra physiotherapy by someone who took me and my HMS seriously. He listened to me thoroughly and for once helped me properly as he understood my condition. I remember feeling so happy and relieved after that first session. It makes such a difference when we come across such a person on our journey. He gave me exercises to do on a daily basis which were very helpful and I've done them until recently. They were very gentle exercises to start with as that's very important for people in chronic pain/with HMS, as we can't handle the exercises normally given to us by most physiotherapists who don't know enough about HMS but often say and think they do!

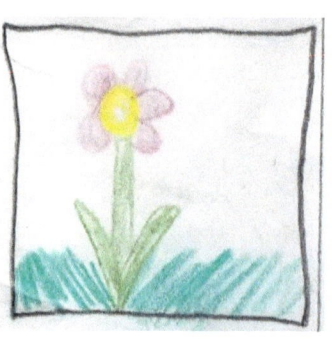

Meanwhile I read up on HMS/chronic pain conditions as a few new books had just been published and I educated myself as much as I could. That's when I realized my husband had HMS too! We never knew, but it then made sense why the kids got it so bad.....he just displayed other symptoms as well such as chest pain, heart palpitations, migraines and repetitive strain injury in his wrist and physical and mental exhaustion. So he went to UCL too and also got diagnosed. He was convinced that a lot of his symptoms were from stress, which certainly can play a big role. We both improved with the help from UCL and especially I embraced it and became 50% better which was huge for me. I was asked by the physio what my end goal was and I said to dance again...but couldn't see it happening, as even walking was hard. A month ago I went to my first session of Bollywood dancing, I can't believe it. I'm so proud of myself and what I've achieved, but I'm getting ahead of myself here.

SUPPORT GROUP

In 2011, I decided to set up a support group in Hampshire for others, as I knew many people needed support like us but there were no support groups in our area when we needed it, which would have made life much easier. So I set one up via the HMSA as they have local support groups all over the country. People came every month and sometimes they came for a private visit and boy was I glad to share my info, knowledge and experience with others who desperately needed it. I saw other friends and families get better with the right help and feeling heard and glad they'd come to the right place to get appropriate information that could help them. For details of local support groups near you (or looking into setting one up if there isn't one in your area) and other valuable information regarding HMS /chronic pain conditions go to HMSA's website listed in the back of this book.

VARIOUS TREATMENTS

Meanwhile I was always looking for further help/cure in the alternative health area, as I had experienced many benefits there. I believe there is more to health than the medical world can provide! Along the way I tried homeopathy, reflexology, acupressure, iridology, chiropractors, physiotherapy, acupuncture, re-birthing (now that was a bit too intense an experience even for me!), healing, reiki, massage, shiatsu, aromatherapy, water aerobics, Pilates, osteopathy, flower remedies, herbal medicine, kinesiology, supplements, magnet therapy, metamorphic technique, visualisation, meditation, breathing techniques, counselling and had my mercury fillings taken out of my teeth.....I was discussing my health issues on the Arnica network forum online (see **Extra Information** section at the back of this book) for months, and eventually was recommended a homeopath/nutritionist who'd had a similar pain condition when young and cured herself via homeopathy and nutrition, by eating a high raw diet and avoiding gluten, meat, dairy and sugar, not overeating, positive thinking and self- talk. So that's what we did and it worked. It was a strict diet and at times very hard to follow but the effects were amazing. I'd never felt so good in years. And the kids can walk to and from school more than a kilometre each way every day now! When we received my daughter's school report after she'd started treatment she suddenly had better marks than ever as she was in less pain and more balanced holistically, so it was easier for her to concentrate. Now she's on par or above her peers which is amazing for us as before she was always below in many subjects so we are very happy. My husband walks one hour every day to and from work. I'd say we are 80- 90% better. The kids are at the same level in everything in life as their peers including health - which is huge!! I'm hoping to get to 95% improvement and then I'll feel normal and feel I've achieved great health for me and my family, and we'll get there...but we are still on a journey to get well even though I feel more and more that I've now reached the goal of healing my family. It took me many years to get this unwell so it might also take quite a while to get well, but boy is it a relief to finally having found something that actually helps so much! I wish everyone had access to this information so they have the opportunity to choose this and get help like we did, hence I'm writing this book for all of you. Because wow if I had acquired this knowledge sooner I would have been thrilled to be able to get well sooner and my kids also, but at least we can now whilst they're still fairly young and hopefully you can too.

ACCESS CONSCIOUSNESS

Since writing the previous chapter, I came across something called Access Consciousness. A healer/body worker gently worked on my head mostly for an hour and cleared old patterns in my body and it's all about learning to listen to and communicate with your body and intuition and positive self-talk. Right away I saw major results! I can now go for several long walks a day, play tennis, dance, run, play with the kids, cook, help out at school and do active hobbies. I'm even writing up my CV for the first time in many years as I'm going to apply for part-time work! I played football on the weekend which I haven't done in 10 years! And I can now eat anything I like! Access Consciousness can work on any aspect of your life. But it's explained much better on their website than I ever could. Please refer to the **Extra Information** section in the back of the book.

HOW TO MAKE IT POSSIBLE FINANCIALLY

Some people have expressed worry over the financial costs using alternative therapies. The way we found worked best for us was to join a health insurance scheme that then covered much of the costs of our treatments. We used the companies Medicash and Simply Health in England (see below for details). We found them very helpful and we didn't have to disclose our medical problems to them.

We emigrated to Australia in September 2012 but we still work with the same practitioner in the UK via Skype as she's helped us so much. We also use Access Consciousness techniques. And what better health insurance to have than to keep my body healthy by listening to it and controlling what I put into it! It's saving us money and we no longer have to go to constant hospital visits, treatments and buy physical aids.

HOW TO OVERCOME CHRONIC PAIN?

When people ask me this question I probably have a different take on it than many. I've always kept searching on the alternative side when 'the medical health care system' gave up on me or couldn't help me many years ago. If I knew then what I know now I'd go straight to my homeopath/nutritionist as she's helped me more in one year - even in the first month - than anything else I've ever done and I've done a lot! Or Access Consciousness as that was also helpful! If people aren't into alternative health there's also help now to get from 'the medical health care system', WHEN/IF you go to the right places where health care professionals are knowledgeable about HMS! My experience was in England so I know UCL and Great Ormond St Hospital are good places to go. These options take time, 'the system' took the longest but for me the outcome was best with the alternative approach. Nevertheless I learned a lot from the hospitals and was very grateful for their help in so many ways at that time. Dietary advice regarding HMS is now sometimes included at UCL and I have spoken to at least one person who was helped a lot by this. So there's hope when the alternative and medical health care worlds merge. I advise you to choose what makes sense to you, take what you can use and adjust it to what works for you.

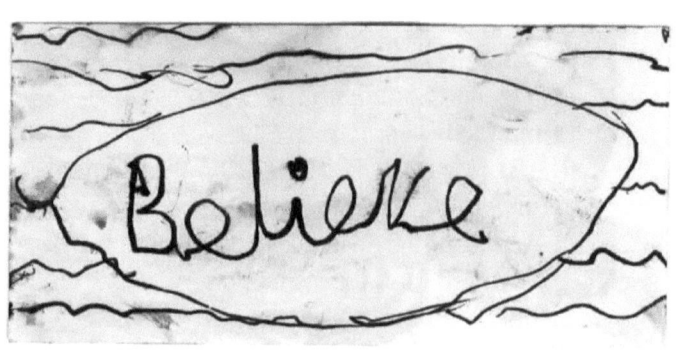

After starting with my UK practitioner within the first month I was 90% better health wise than I'd ever been. She had us doing hair tests to find out the levels of heavy metals in our systems, which can cause a lot of harm if you have high levels. And we did. We all had very high levels of arsenic which might be from pesticides and chemicals being sprayed on crops in conventional farming and ingesting it via the crops or in the air. That could well be the case with me as I grew up on a conventional farm. I could have also passed it on to the kids when pregnant.

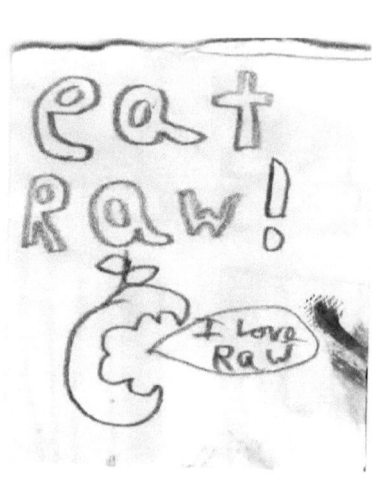

I can't say I have the answers for what can heal everyone as everyone's different! I believe different things work for different people! But what I want to do with this book is to let you know that I believe it's possible for people with a chronic pain condition to get better, if you keep searching for alternatives and trying things that resonate with you. I can't even say what exactly healed me but maybe a combination of all the above! Don't give up - I believe there is a way of healing for all of us!

Healing thoughts to you on your journey,

Storm:)

EXTRA INFORMATION:

My email address in case of additional questions or comments:
storm.furness@yahoo.com.au

WEBSITES

HMSA website: www.hypermobility.org has lots of valuable resources re. HMS and Chronic pain disorders including local support groups in UK and an online forum to chat to people in a similar situation as you. They also sell books on HMS and more and send you newsletters if you become a member.

www.arnica.org.uk is a website based in the UK, set up less than a decade ago by a mother who wished to spread more awareness of natural immunity. It has relevant worldwide information on holistic health and natural immunity with a forum where anyone can ask questions and discuss health issues. There are also local Arnica support groups mainly in UK but also now abroad.

BOOKS

Douglas, G. M. (2012) *Right body for You*. Littleton, USA: Big Country Publishing, LLC.
He is the founder of Access Consciousness.

HEALTH INSURANCE (UK only listed - but I know there are similar in Australia and other countries):

Simply Health

Medicash

PRACTITIONERS

Dawn Waterhouse, homeopath, nutritionist, UK,
www.dawnwaterhouse.co.uk

Access Consciousness (on their website you can find
practitioners in your area), Australia and worldwide,
www.accessconsciousness.com